Return to Play

Guide to the Mental Aspects of Rehabilitation for Injured Athletes

Kathleen Kickish, MS, ATC, LAT

Abbott Press books may be ordered through booksellers or by contacting:

Abbott Press
1663 Liberty Drive
Bloomington, IN 47403
www.abbottpress.com
Phone: 1-866-697-5310

Because of the dynamic nature of the Internet, any web addresses or links contained in this book may have changed since publication and may no longer be valid. The views expressed in this work are solely those of the author and do not necessarily reflect the views of the publisher, and the publisher hereby disclaims any responsibility for them.

Any people depicted in stock imagery provided by Thinkstock are models, and such images are being used for illustrative purposes only.

Certain stock imagery © Thinkstock.

ISBN: 978-1-4582-1015-9 (sc)
ISBN: 978-1-4582-1014-2 (e)

Printed in the United States of America.

Abbott Press rev. date: 06/13/13

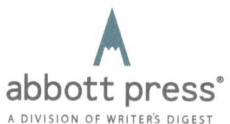

abbott press®
A DIVISION OF WRITER'S DIGEST

This book is dedicated to all of the injured athletes reading it that are willing and motivated enough to do whatever it takes to put in the maximal effort mentally and physically to return to their sport at their fullest capacity. Your dedication and drive continually motivate and inspire others.

Letter to the Injured Athlete

Dear Athlete,

Welcome to your very own guide through the mental aspects of rehabilitation from injury, better known as the **psychological rehabilitation process**. First, it is very important for you to recognize that an injury does not only affect you physically, but there is also a mental, or psychological, component that must be identified and properly addressed. You must think of yourself as a whole person, and rehabilitation as an integrated process taking care of **all** aspects of you. You may be going through a whole series of emotions and feelings right now as a result of your injury including, but not limited to, anger, guilt, helplessness, fear, frustration, depression, and uncertainty. It is important for you to understand that all of these reactions and emotions are completely normal and to keep changing from one feeling to another is also normal. These responses are physical as well as psychological and how you respond to your injury is unique to you.

This book will help you to learn more about yourself as well as the psychological aspects that may affect your rehabilitation process and how to deal with them in the most effective way. It is constructed in a way that it should help you to better understand what is happening to you both mentally and physically. It will help you to understand what your role is in rehabilitation and will serve as a supplement to the physical rehabilitation you are currently undergoing. Additionally, this book will help you to recognize and assess certain characteristics about yourself, such as personality type, and how these characteristics impact both your psychological and physical rehabilitation processes.

Throughout the book, numerous questions are posed. At these points, stop and ask yourself those questions, write down your answers, and reflect on the responses you have given. It is strongly recommended to keep a journal of some sort. Whether you use a notebook, a computer, or a formal journal, use whatever works best for you, as long as you make it something that is **yours**. This technique will help by allowing you a specified place to write down your answers to the questions posed as well as to keep an account of your feelings and thoughts in regard to your injury and your journey through rehabilitation. By writing these things down in a specific place, it will allow you to go back and reflect upon your answers as well as previous answers and feelings.

This book will furthermore help you to evaluate your responses to the questions posed and take appropriate action in order to engage in the most effective rehabilitation. It may also help to discuss some of these answers with your athletic trainer, physical therapist, or other health care professional. This is encouraged because they are often the individuals who have the most frequent contact with you during your physical rehabilitation and are educated in some aspects of psychological rehabilitation. In addition, it may be beneficial for you to seek the services of a sport psychologist. There is a page in the back of this book that will give you tips on how to contact a sport psychologist if you would like to talk to one. Lastly, this book offers various techniques to try in order to assess your own psychological response to injury and how to most effectively handle, or cope with, this response. Following this guide and learning how to most effectively handle your personal psychological response to injury will help you to return to your sport, ready to play both physically and psychologically.

Sincerely,

Kathleen Kickish, MS, ATC, LAT

Table of Contents

Chapter 1:

Your Roles

In Rehabilitation

Your Roles in Rehabilitation:

It is beneficial for you to first identify what your specific roles are in the rehabilitation process. Listen to your health care professional and follow their specific instructions in order to restore your health and function as quickly and safely as possible. The following includes some of your personal roles in rehabilitation as the injured athlete. Pay close attention as these are **your** roles.

- Educate yourself about your injury and the rehabilitation process.
  - Ask your athletic trainer, physical therapist, doctor, or other health care professional to help educate you about your specific injury and help you to find credible resources for information from books, journal articles, and **reliable** internet sources.
  - Ask questions! Those that do not ask questions will never get answers. If there is anything that you are unclear or uncertain about, ask.
  - Educate your coach, teammates, and family by sharing the information with them about your injury and your process through rehabilitation.
- Stay involved with the team.
  - Keep your coaches up to date with your progress by communicating with them regularly.
  - Seek social support through your team during rehabilitation to help stay involved with your sport.
  - Consult with your coaches on finding ways to stay involved with the team other than playing on the field (examples include taking statistics, helping with

equipment, handing out water, helping with drills in practice, and spending time with teammates outside of the sport atmosphere).

- o Identify what ways to stay involved work best for you personally and are beneficial to your team and coach.

- Be devoted to the rehabilitation protocol set by your health care professional.

  - o Take responsibility for rehabilitation. This is **your** rehabilitation.

  - o Show up on time and ready to work.

  - o Complete all home exercises. Perform these exercises the specified number of times and for the specified duration that you are instructed.

  - o Take rehabilitation seriously and put in **optimal** effort.

    - Listen to your athletic trainer and do not "over-do-it" or "under-do-it". Optimal effort for your stage of recovery is key.

    - Listen to your body and what it is telling you during rehabilitation to see if you are pushing it too far or if you can push it more.

    - Be consistent! Consistency is key to a fast and safe recovery.

- Have a positive attitude.

  - o Have confidence in yourself and your ability to recover.

  - o Avoid a negative attitude. Negative attitudes may impede the psychological, as well as physical, rehabilitation process.

  - o Recognize when you are displaying a negative attitude or have a negative frame of mind and try to reframe your thoughts as well as your words to display a positive attitude.

- Seek support.

  - o If you do not seek it, you will not get it.

- Parents, siblings, friends, coaches, classmates, teammates, significant others, all can be part of your support network and can provide support in different ways.

- Prioritize rehabilitation!
  - You will get out of it as much as you put into it. If you want to get back to the same level of play you were at before your injury or at an even higher level, make rehabilitation a top priority in your life.

- Set realistic goals and expectations, both short-term and long-term.
  - Work with your athletic trainer or other health care professional to set short-term and long-term rehabilitation goals. Talk to these individuals about what is realistic and what is not as well as steps to take to achieve these goals.

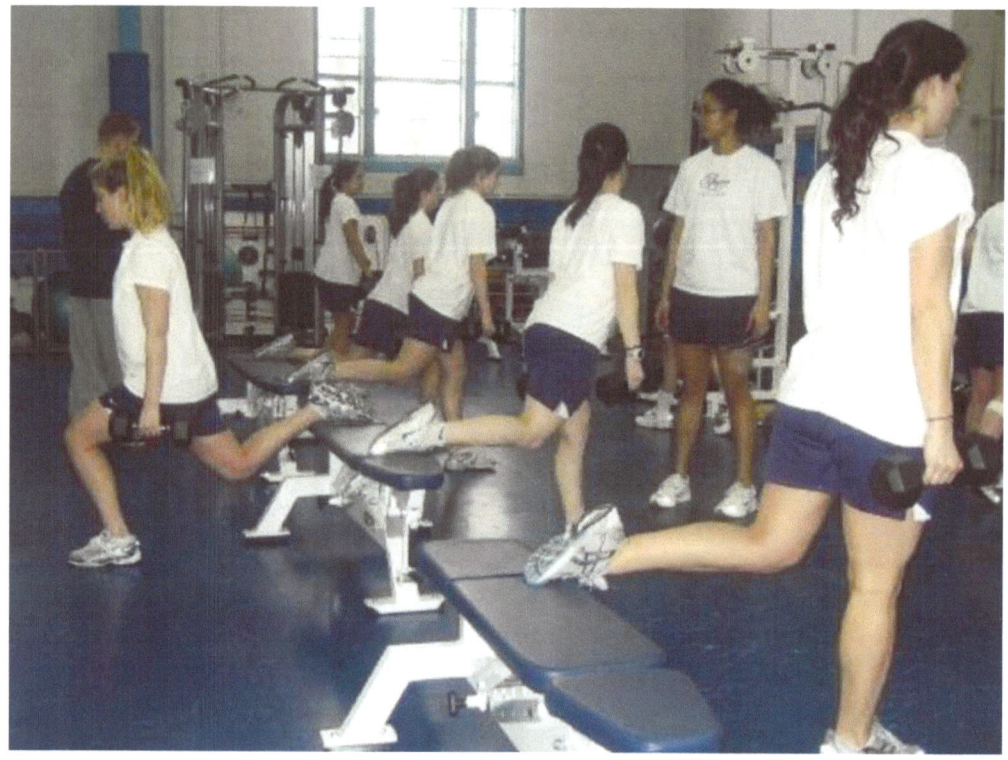

Take Responsibility For Your Rehabilitation

What you can control and what you can NOT control in your rehabilitation:

These factors are very important to keep in mind. As much as you want to be able to control everything, you must realize that some things are out of your control. Accepting this fact is an important step in rehabilitation from injury. Below is a list of things that you can control in your rehabilitation and another list of things that may be beyond your control as you progress through rehabilitation.

What you can control:

- Your attitude toward and perception of pain

- Your activities outside of rehabilitation

- Work ethic, motivation, and positive thinking

- Taking personal responsibility for your rehabilitation

- Having realistic expectations

- Being devoted to your rehabilitation in the athletic training room and at home

- Educating yourself about your injury and asking questions for clarification

- Having confidence in yourself during rehabilitation and having confidence in the fact that you will recover fully

- How you view yourself and your identity through self-perception

- Your personal reactions to injury and rehabilitation

- Trusting and having confidence in your athletic trainer or other health care professional

What you can NOT control:

- What the team does while you are injured

- Physical environment surrounding you during rehabilitation

- How long your recovery will take
    - However, you can influence it by being devoted to your rehabilitation routine, putting in optimal effort during rehabilitation, following the psychological techniques outlined in this manual, and listening carefully to the directions of your health care professional

- What other people do during the duration of your rehabilitation such as coaches, teammates, friends, and family

- How other people perceive you and react towards you and your injury

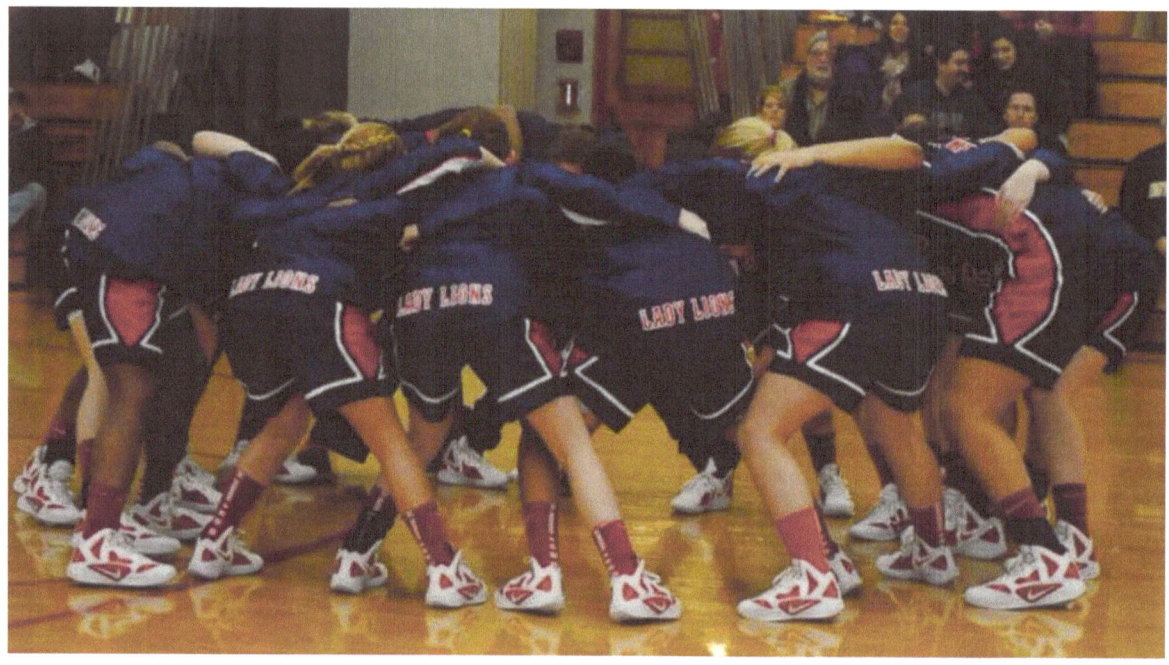

Chapter 2:

Personality and

Self-Identity

Personality and Self- Identity

It is very important to recognize and assess your own personality traits; including assessing your self-identity, evaluating your level of athletic identity, and determining how these factors may affect your rehabilitation process both physically and psychologically. **Self-identity** is how you personally perceive yourself and define yourself as an individual. Make sure to think of yourself as a whole person with many dimensions and take into consideration how your injury may be affecting other parts of your life such as school, family, friends, work, and other relationships. Take the time now to reflect on what personality characteristics you see in yourself to help assess your self-identity. Look at examples in the chart on page 20 if you need help getting started. Ask yourself the questions below, write down your answers, and reflect on what your answers may say about your self-identity.

1. **What defining personality characteristics do you see in yourself?**

2. **How do you feel others view you? Does this affect how you view yourself?**

3. **How do you view your self-identity? What aspects of your life define you?**

4. **What words would you use to describe yourself and your roles in life?**

5. **What percentage of yourself do you feel is defined by being an athlete?**

6. **What other activities or hobbies are you involved in besides your sport?**

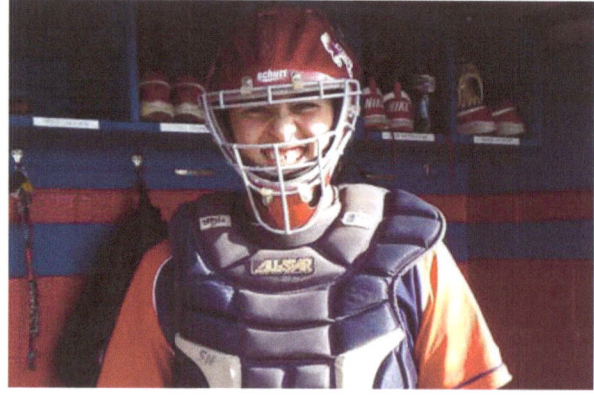

Athletic Identity

What aspects or roles of your life do you believe define you as a person? **Athletic identity** is defined as the degree to which individuals identify with their role as an athlete and use this identification to define who they are as a person as well as give them a sense of self-worth (Griffith & Johnson, 2002). There are some good aspects of an athlete having a high athletic identity, such as dedication to the team and the sport. However, when individuals with a high athletic identity become injured, it may become a problem because they may feel like a part of them is missing.

Do you feel that being injured has changed your self-identity?

It is important to measure your personal perceived athletic identity by asking yourself how much you believe being an athlete defines you. To measure your own athletic identity, please ask yourself the questions below, think sincerely about the questions as well as your answers, and write down your responses. After you are finished, reflect on your answers and assess what they may say about your athletic identity, or to what degree you define your self-identity as an athlete. You should discuss these with your athletic trainer, other health care professional, or sport psychologist to help gauge your athletic identity if you feel comfortable.

1. **What percentage of your day does sport take up? (This includes playing prior to your injury, thinking about it, discussing it with friends, etc.)**

2. **What are your goals in life? Are they related to sport? Are these realistic goals? How many of your goals are related to being an athlete?**

3. **Are most of your friends athletes? If so, are they on the same sports team as you or on a different sports team?**

4. How important is it to you to be an athlete? Why?

5. What is the most important aspect of your life? Why?

6. Has being injured affected who you are? If so, how?

7. How much of your day is spent thinking about sports in general (such a professional sports in addition to your own sport)?

8. Does how you perform in your sport affect how you feel about yourself?

9. How would you feel if you could no longer play your sport? How do you think this would affect your life?

Below is an example of an individual's perceived self-identity. Think of yourself as a whole pie and each one of the roles you identify with as slices of that pie. As you may notice, the greatest portion of this male individual's self-identity he defines as being an athlete. This **may** become a problem because he defines himself more as an athlete than he does as a family member.

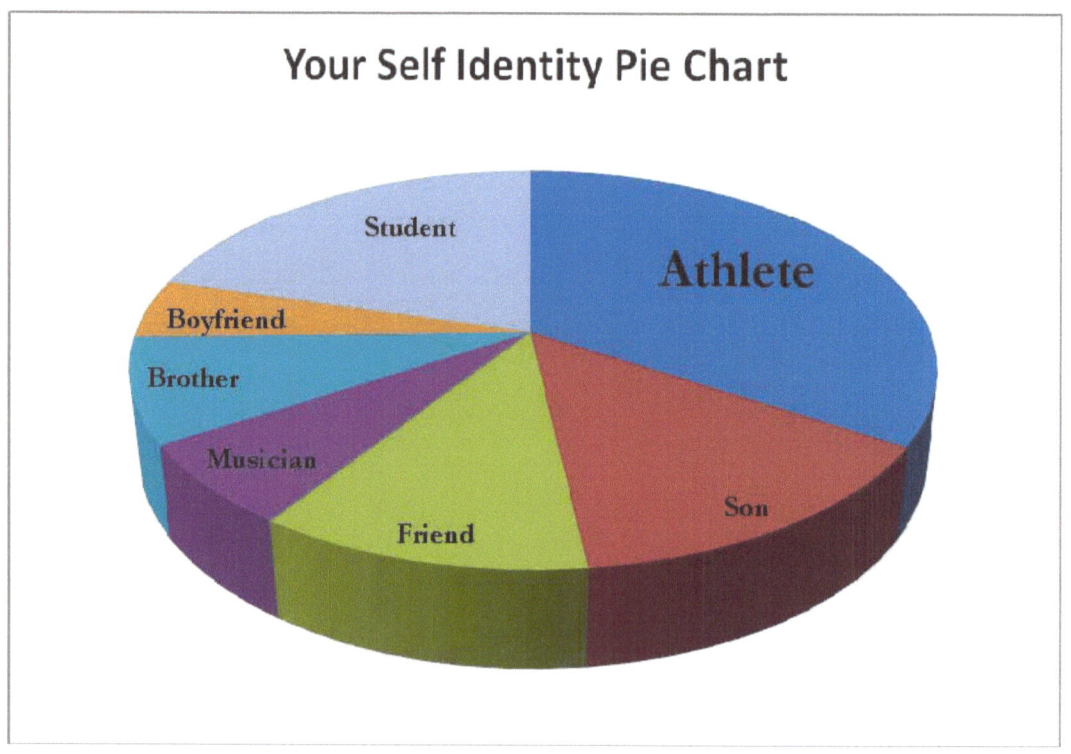

Maintaining Athletic Identity

It is also important for you to try to maintain your personal level of athletic identity throughout rehabilitation. With the help of your athletic trainer or other rehabilitation professional, you may incorporate many things into the rehabilitation process to maintain your own sense of athletic identity and stay involved with the team. Other items you can do at home or outside of the rehabilitation setting. Such items include but are not limited to:

- View rehabilitation as a form of athletic performance

- Perform rehabilitation exercises on the sidelines during practices

- Use performance imagery to mentally "practice" your athletic skills in your mind by closing your eyes and mentally going through the motions that you would while playing your sport

- Have regular meetings with the coach and stay informed about the team as well as to keep the coach informed about your progress in rehabilitation.

- Stay involved with and help the team by doing things such as recording statistics, helping take care of equipment, videotaping, or aiding the coach in observations of the team

- Engage in other forms of physical activity that are safe to perform with your injury

- Socialize with teammates outside of sport situations

- Be in the locker room before and after practices and games

- Travel to games with the team when possible

- Use positive self-talk when speaking about your injury and in rehabilitation

- Use sport specific functional exercises, or similar movements and exercises that you might use in your sport, in your physical rehabilitation process as designated by your athletic trainer or other health care professional

- Focus on the present and the future, not the past

What other techniques can you use to maintain your athletic identity and stay involved with the team? Write these down in your journal and try to incorporate them into your life and rehabilitation. Identify which ones work best for you!

Personality Type Check- List Worksheet

Use this table to check-off the personality characteristics that you may see in yourself. Put an X or check-mark next to the characteristics that you feel you possess. After you are finished, move on to the next page to read what your answers may say about your own personality, how you respond to stress, and how these characteristics may affect rehabilitation.

	Check List		Check List		Check List
Competitive		Relaxed		Easy-Going	
Friendly		Eager to Please		Compliant	
Energetic		Patient		Driven (highly motivated)	
Respectful		Flexible		Laid-Back	
Controlling		Introverted		Gives up when there is a high amount of stress	
Conforming		Easy to please		Dependant on others	
Independent		Impatient		Ambitious	

Personality Types

There are various outlined personality types that individuals may identify with. Three main classified **personality types** are type A, type B, and type C. Due to the characteristics of the personality types, you may be at risk in rehabilitation for over-adherence or under-adherence, (i.e., "over-doing-it" or "under-doing-it"), depending with which personality type you identify. A brief description of these personality types and the possible effects they may have on your health and rehabilitation process are listed below:

(Table adapted from: Susic, 1999)

Personality Type	Characteristics of Type
Type A	competitive, impatient, energetic, driven, controlling, and ambitious, independent
Type B	takes life more slowly, relaxed, laid back, easy-going, patient, friendly, easy to please, flexible
Type C	responds to stress by giving up, introverted, respectful, eager to please, conforming and compliant, dependant on others

Type A individuals, due to their impatient, hardworking, and driven personality, may be at risk for over-adherence in an attempt to speed up the process of rehabilitation and complete it as quickly as possible. They tend to believe that the harder they work, and the more they do, the faster they will recover. However, this is a false assumption. Over-adherence means that individuals will try to do too much during rehabilitation, beyond what they are instructed to do. This behavior has a risk of further injuring the athlete or causing a new injury.

Conversely, individuals with type B personality may be at risk for under-adherence due to their laid back and relaxed personality. This type of individual may not get enough out of rehabilitation or the rehabilitation may take longer because the individual does not put in enough effort. You may be type B if you come in to rehabilitation only when you feel like it and do not come in when you simply do not want to or come in late. Type B individuals may also have a tendency to skip their home rehabilitation exercises. These behaviors are a sign that you do not make rehabilitation a priority. As you can imagine, this is a significant problem, as rehabilitation should be a top priority in order to fully recover.

Type C personality may be prone to either over-adhere or under-adhere depending on which aspects of their personality are more dominant. If you respond to stress in your life with depression and hopelessness, you may feel hopeless about rehabilitation and thus feel like your effort does not matter. Therefore, you may be at risk for under-adherence in your rehabilitation. On the other hand, if you have a strong desire to please others and be compliant, you may be at risk for over-adherence. It is important to recognize and assess your individual personality type as well as defining characteristics that may affect rehabilitation and respond in ways that will facilitate recovery.

Look back at your answers from the personality type work-sheet that you filled out. Reflect on your own personality characteristics outlined in the table as well as other personality characteristics that you see in yourself that may not have been mentioned. Determine how these characteristics may affect your rehabilitation process and how you feel toward rehabilitation. Write down in your journal how you feel about these characteristics and how you can actively try to acknowledge and modify characteristics that may negatively affect rehabilitation in order to have a more effective experience

Chapter 3:

Cognitive

Appraisal

Cognitive Appraisal

Cognitive appraisal is how individuals mentally evaluate and perceive a certain situation or event in their life (Brough & Oliver, 2002). It is important for you to reflect on and evaluate your own subjective experience of your injury and the rehabilitation process. Subjective means how <u>you</u> personally evaluate what is going on and observe your environment or situation as opposed to how another person may evaluate it, in which case it would be objective.

Injury may evoke many emotional and psychological responses in an athlete. The range of these responses may vary in how each individual experiences them, but many can be compared to the five stages of grief originally outlined by psychologist Elizabeth Kubler-Ross. These stages are a progression of psychological and emotional reactions that athletes may have to injury or any other hardship in their life. The outlined progression of these responses includes denial, anger, bargaining, depression, and acceptance (Kubler-Ross, 1969). While often the reactions are experienced in this order, you may experience them in a different order, skip stages, or revert back to previous reactions. All of these progressions are normal and how you experience them depends on your personal cognitive appraisal of the injury.

Commonly the first psychological reaction to injury in the athlete is denial. Athletes may deny that anything is wrong with them, or deny the extent of their injury and try to go about their daily life normally, as if they did not have an injury. This can be detrimental as it may place the athletes at risk for additional injury if they go beyond what their injury physically allows them to do. The next reaction of the progression is typically anger. This may be anger at themselves for becoming injured, anger at the nature of the sport itself, or displaced anger on any other object or individual. As you can imagine, this reaction can negatively impact rehabilitation immensely. Following anger, the injured individuals usually go into the phase of bargaining. With this reaction, athletes will often try to speed their recovery process by attempting to bargain, or make deals, with their health care professional, coach, or any other person that may have an influence on their return to play. A typical bargaining response may be, "if I do all of my exercises every day for two weeks, can I play in the next game?" When athletes do not get the response from these individuals that they want, they may go into the next progressive stage, depression. In this stage, athletes may become withdrawn or hopeless about their recovery. They may begin to feel sorry for themselves and feel as if they want to give up trying to recover. This stage has a tendency to impede rehabilitation by the individuals not putting optimal effort into rehabilitation due to their hopelessness. The most important transition is between this reaction and the next, acceptance. With the reaction of acceptance, athletes acknowledge the fact that they are injured and that they must go through physical rehabilitation as well as put in optimal effort in order to recover and return to their sport.

The range of reactions you are experiencing as a result of your injury, both physical as well as psychological, are unique to you in how you experience them. However, it is extremely important that you recognize that all of these reactions are completely normal. Acknowledge what you are experiencing and be conscious of it. Express these feelings by writing them down. It may be beneficial for you to speak with a sport psychologist or other licensed professional about how you feel about the injury and rehabilitation process. Ask yourself the questions below, write down your answers in full detail, and reflect on your responses:

- How does your injury make you feel?

- Is your injury affecting other aspects of your life? If so, how?

- How do you feel about your rehabilitation process?

- What aspects of your rehabilitation are working for you? What aspects are not?

- How can your rehabilitation process work better for you?

Integrative Process of Subjective Assessment

It is important for you to identify and approach the personal, social, psychological, and physical factors that may be affecting the rehabilitation process and recognize how these factors integrate, relate to, and affect each other. This is a holistic process, meaning it affects you as a whole person. You may assess yourself on personal, social, psychological, and physical factors by reflecting on your strengths and weaknesses in these areas. These factors of your rehabilitation may be assessed to determine how you feel you are progressing or not progressing during rehabilitation. Take a look at the factors on the following pages and consider how strong or weak you personally perceive and interpret yourself in each area. Revisit this page and your answers approximately **once a week or once every other week** as you progress in your rehabilitation. Determine which areas become stronger or weaker as you progress. These subjective assessments, in addition to observations by your athletic trainer or other rehabilitation professional, complete a compilation that can be used to assess different perspectives on the complete integrated rehabilitation process.

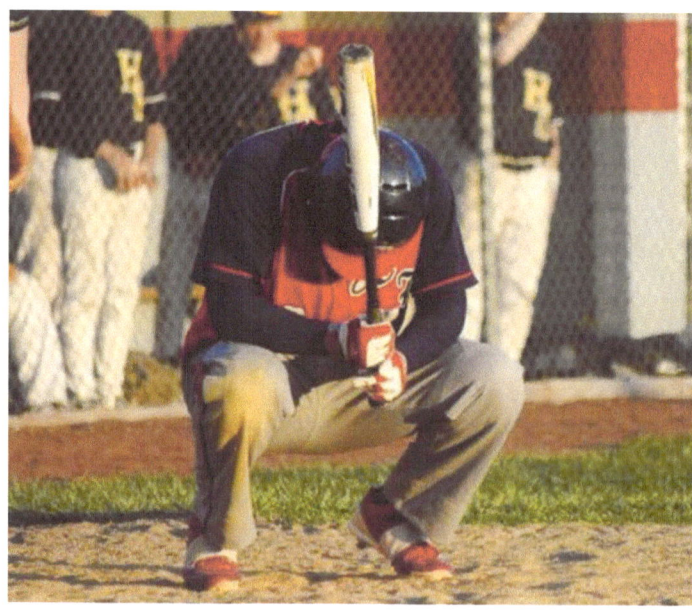

Cognitive Appraisal Worksheet

Consider how strong or weak you perceive yourself in the following areas- place an X on the weak-strong continuum to assess where you think you stand. Record your answers and discuss them with your athletic trainer, sport psychologist, or other health care professional. Fill it out once a week or once every other week during the rehabilitation process to see how you are cognitively progressing.

(Table adapted from: Taylor & Taylor, 1997)

Physical Factors:	Weak---Strong
Muscle Strength	Weak---Strong
Stability of Joint	Weak---Strong
Coordination	Weak---Strong
Balance	Weak---Strong
Swelling (a little or a lot?)	Weak---Strong
Pain (a little or a lot?)	Weak---Strong
Range of Motion of Injured Area	Weak---Strong
Fatigue	Weak---Strong
Function of Injured Area	Weak---Strong
Overall Health	Weak---Strong
Sleeping	Weak---Strong

Psychological, Personal, and Social Factors:	Weak--Strong
Anxiety	Weak--Strong
Focus	Weak--Strong
Worry	Weak--Strong
Guilt	Weak--Strong
Anger	Weak--Strong
Understanding	Weak--Strong
Motivation	Weak--Strong
Fear	Weak--Strong
Social Support	Weak--Strong
Hopelessness	Weak--Strong
Determination	Weak--Strong
Adherence to Rehabilitation Protocol	Weak--Strong
Athletic Identity	Weak--Strong

- Additionally, write in your journal or other specified area:

    o How do you feel about your responses? What do you think your feelings say about your reaction to injury and rehabilitation?

    o Are you surprised at your answers?

    o How are your answers different from previous weeks?

    o What emotions are you feeling?

    o What are your expectations for rehabilitation?

Chapter 4:

Stress

And

Burnout

Stress and Burnout

Many outside factors and events in your life may be affecting your rehabilitation process. Whether you are aware of it or not, all aspects of your life interact and impact each other. Again, you must look at yourself as a whole person with many integrated parts. You should recognize that other aspects of your life, such as stressful life events, may be causing you additional stress and, therefore, may be affecting the physical and psychological rehabilitation process or your personal response to your injury. Whether you are experiencing **eustress**, also known as positive stress, or **distress**, defined as negative stress, it puts the same physiological stress on the body and mind. Examples of eustress may be the birth of a new baby in the family or an upcoming wedding while examples of distress may be the death of a loved one or the divorce of parents, depending on how you personally perceive these situations. This additional stress can possibly lead to a term called "burnout," which is complete exhaustion physically or emotionally, usually as a result of prolonged stress, which leads to deterioration of physical functions and impairment of the immune system (Fevre, Kolt, & Matheny, 2003). This will significantly impede your rehabilitation.

On the next page, there are some examples of stressful events and circumstances you may be experiencing that may be causing you significant stress and may therefore be negatively affecting your rehabilitation process. Examine this list and identify which items you are currently experiencing in your life, or which have occurred to you recently. Consider how these events or circumstances may be placing additional stress on you, especially in a cumulative manner, and affecting your rehabilitation. Also, consider how you may, with this knowledge, combat the stress these circumstances are adding to your life by identifying how you may cope, or deal with, them.

Examples of Life Stressors

(Table adapted from: Holmes & Rahe, 1967)

Death of someone close to you	Increased responsibility in your life
Parents' divorce or separation	Health problem of a family member or someone close to you
Puberty	Being fired from work or expelled from school
Pregnancy	Change in personal financial status or that of parents
Getting in trouble with the law	Working while attending school
Engagement	Transfer of schools
Getting in trouble in school	Moving or relocation
Personal illness	Change in relationship status with significant other such as a breakup or a new relationship
Beginning the next level of school (example: from high school to college)	Bad test grades or poor performance in school
Substance use or abuse (drugs or alcohol)	Change in or problem with friends
Lack of sleep or trouble sleeping	Parent remarried
Death or illness of pet	Getting a new pet
Change in appearance (ex: getting braces)	Birth of sibling or someone in family
Vacation	New job

- What is the most significant source of stress in your life, whether it is eustress (positive) or distress (negative)? Why?

- If possible, how can you make this area less stressful?

- In your journal identify the main sources of stress in your life and rank them by those that produce the most stress and those that produce the least stress. Then, identify at least 2-3 ways each to make those producing the most stress less stressful

31

If one or more of these stressful events or circumstances have happened to you recently, you may be at risk for additional stress on top of the stress your current injury is placing on your life depending on how you view the event and how it has impacted your life. The greater the amount of these stressors that you have experienced, the greater the risk of significant stress, which may cause additional injury or illness. Take time to reflect on how these events or situations have impacted your life, your character, and your rehabilitation, as well as how you personally can cope with this added stress. It may be beneficial for you to see a licensed psychologist or sport psychologist to discuss how these factors have had an impact on you. In the next section of this book, you will find some relaxation and coping techniques that can help you better manage stress, including the stress of your injury.

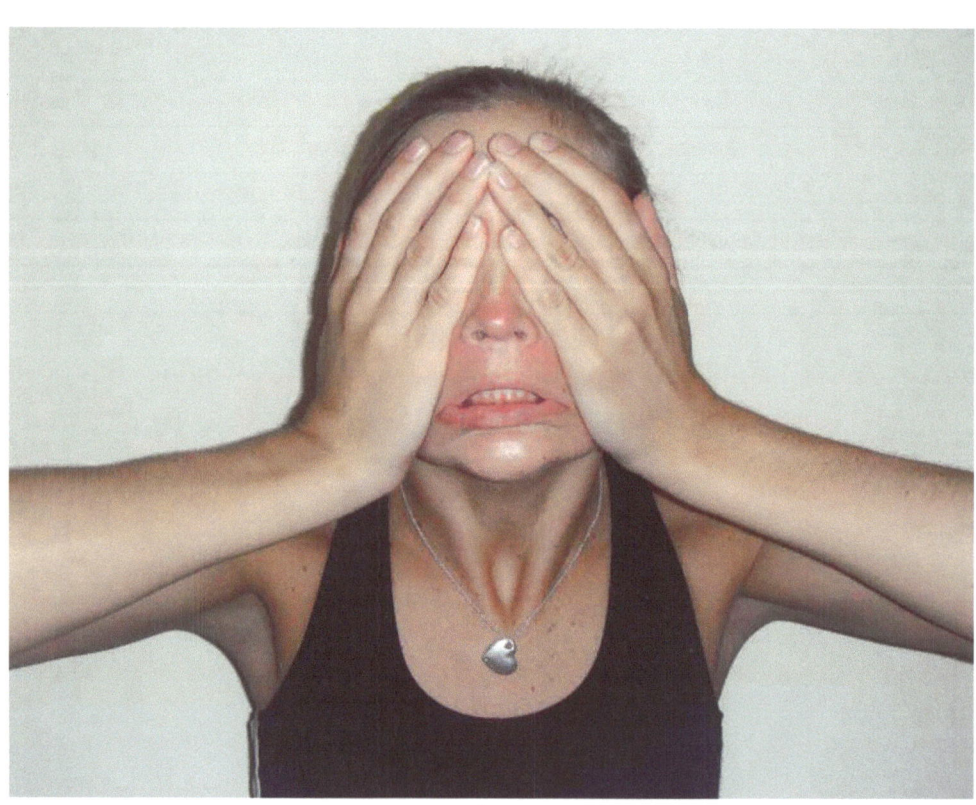

What Stressors Are Impacting Your Life?

Chapter 5:

Psychological

Interventions

Psychological Interventions

There are many things that you personally can do to facilitate and improve your psychological rehabilitation process as well as cope with stress. It is very important that you are motivated and take a lead role in your own physical rehabilitation along with taking control of making your psychological rehabilitation a priority. Increasing your self-efficacy, or your own perceived ability in a task, and self-confidence, or your certainty in yourself, your thoughts, and your abilities, are a large part of the psychological rehabilitation process. Ways in which you can improve in these areas this include the following:

- **Positive self-talk**

- **Negative thought stopping**

- **Actively seeking social support**

- **Goal setting**

- **Relaxation techniques**

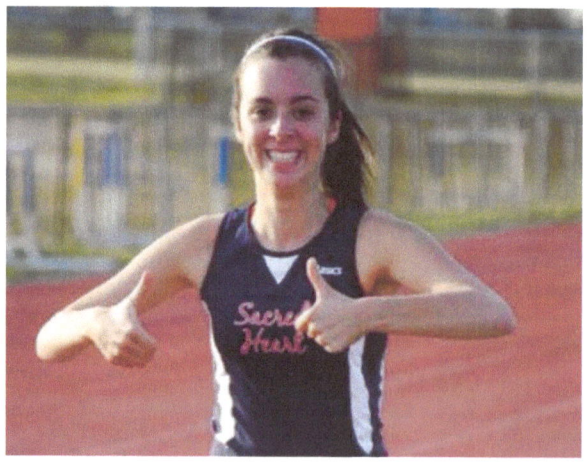

Increasing Self-Confidence Through Positive Self-Talk and Negative Thought Stopping

Self-Confidence is a vital component to rehabilitation and to recovery. If you are not confident in yourself, you will not be able to fully recover and return to your sport effectively. Injured athletes have a tendency to focus on negative elements of their injury and not believe in themselves that they can and will fully recover. By having this negative attitude and ignoring the rehabilitative aspects that are occurring, you impede your own recovery process. Refer back to your self-perceived strengths and weaknesses in the cognitive appraisal section to determine your own level of self-confidence in various areas and to identify what aspects you feel that you need to improve. Talk to your athletic trainer or other health care professional about how to strengthen these factors and thus increase self-confidence.

Positive self-talk is defined as the positive affirmations people say to themselves about their current situation and perceived outcome. It has been shown to be extremely beneficial in terms of increasing an injured athlete's self-confidence level and, in turn, aiding in the psychological rehabilitation process. This technique works best when combined with **negative thought stopping**. Negative thought stopping involves the acknowledgement of a negative thought being formed, and actively stopping yourself from forming the thought or completing a negative statement. (Taylor & Taylor, 1997). When combining these two techniques you stop the negative thoughts and replace them with positive self-talk. A technique to accomplish this is as follows on the next page.

Positive Self- Talk and Negative Thought Stopping Technique

- When you start thinking of something negative, acknowledge it as negative and immediately think of a stop sign (or another effective meaningful symbol that will help stop your thought). Then, actively reframe your words into a positive thought instead of a negative thought.
  - Example: Negative thought= "I cannot complete the 20 wall slides prescribed to me for rehabilitation by my athletic trainer"
  - When the thought begins, acknowledge the thought and think of a stop sign (or another meaningful image). Then reframe the thought to say "I can complete 20 wall slides and will do it to the best of my ability."
- Seek help from those around you and from your social support network to aid you in recognizing when you are thinking or saying something negative. Then, verbalize your positive self-talk back to this individual by rephrasing your statement out loud.
- Practice, practice, practice! The more you practice this technique, the more natural it will become. Positive thoughts lead to positive results.

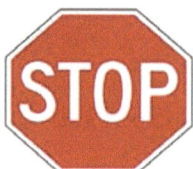

Positive Self-talk and Thought Stopping Worksheet

Use the form below to track your negative self-talk as well as your effort in thought stopping and reframing those thoughts into positive self-talk:

Negative Self-Talk	Thought Stopping Symbol or person who helped you	Reframed Positive Self-Talk

Now, in your journal, write down various ways in which you can increase your positive self-talk and decrease your negative self-talk. Make sure to acknowledge your own progression and improvements in having a more positive outlook on your rehabilitation as you utilize the techniques.

Social Support

Social support is another very beneficial component of rehabilitation. It provides you, the injured athlete, with a sense of interpersonal connectedness and promotes communication between you and other people involved in your life or with your rehabilitation process. Social support shows you that you are not alone in the injury rehabilitation process and that others are there to provide comfort, support, encouragement, and information. With social support, athletes experience greater self-efficacy and self-confidence, better stress management, decreased anxiety, and possibly faster recovery times.

Social support can be provided by anyone and can be provided in numerous ways. For example, you can seek social support through either listening social support or emotional social support. The difference between the two is that with listening social support the individual who is supporting you listens actively and openly to you without judgment or interruption and lets you vent. With emotional social support the individual who is supporting you not only listens to you but also offers encouragement and emotional support with words or actions (Taylor & Taylor, 1997). In this circumstance, the individual offering emotional social support may encourage and challenge you to overcome obstacles and fulfill specified goals or may just offer empathetic support through words and actions. Additionally, you may seek support through a knowledgeable resource, such as your athletic trainer or other health care professional, to gain educational information about your injury. This individual can offer support by relieving your worries and tensions about your injury through educational, or informational, support. They can also offer you praise or positive attention when you accomplish a certain goal or task in your rehabilitation (Taylor & Taylor, 1997). A single person can not help you with all of the social support that you need. You must seek it from multiple diverse sources to fulfill your needs.

It is not essential that the person offering you social support has had similar experiences to you and knows first hand what you are going through. Instead, it is more important that they openly engage with you and try to empathize by offering you their full attention while you are seeking their support. It is imperative that you **actively** seek social support in order to maintain psychological well-being throughout the rehabilitation process. Those that do not seek social support will not get it. You must actively take responsibility for seeking it. Identify on the next page the types of social support that are or can be provided to you. Additionally, identify sources that offer these various types of support to you or could possibly offer these types of support to you, how they make you feel, and whether they are effective in fulfilling your need. Use additional paper if necessary or record responses in your journal.

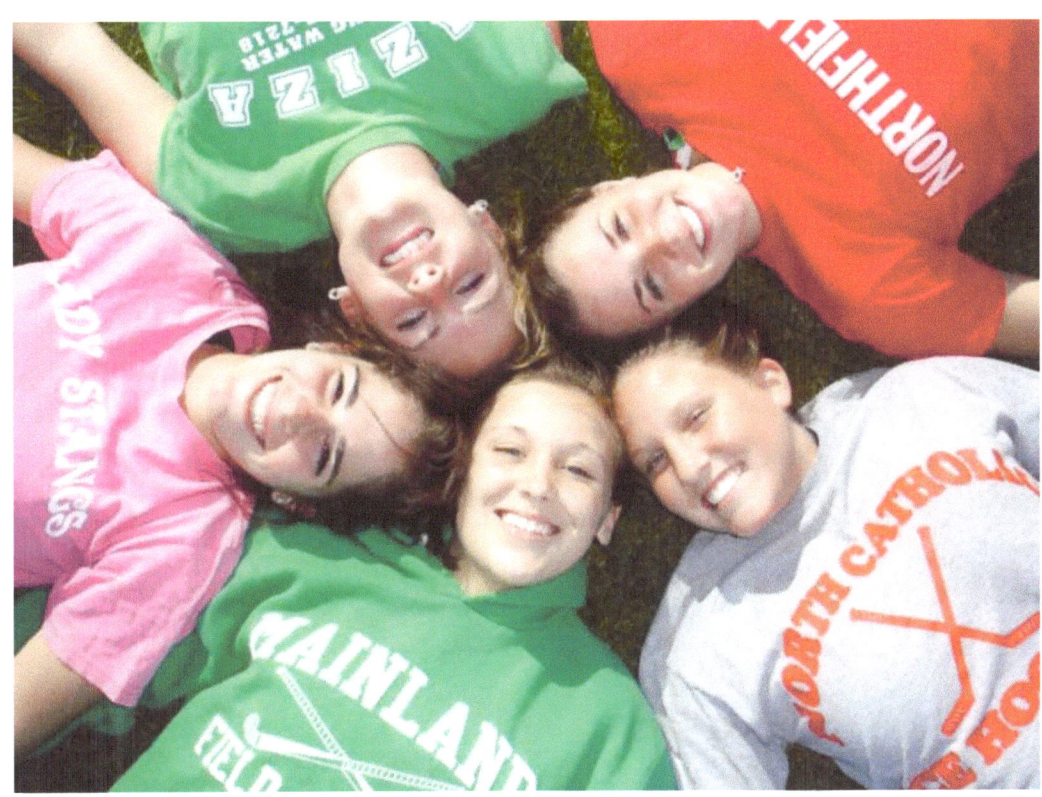

Social Support Work Sheet

Type of Social Support	Source of Social Support (specific person)	How This Type of Support Makes Me Feel (if already provided to you)	Effective in fulfilling my need? If not, how could it be more effective?

Feel free to write additional thoughts in your journal about your sources of social support and how they make you feel. Be sure to also include social support from sources that you do not currently have but that you wish you had and how you can actively seek social support from these sources.

Goal Setting

     Goal setting is an important component in increasing your self-confidence and your self-perceived ability in a task. It helps you to take an active role in the design and implementation of your rehabilitation program by working with your athletic trainer or other qualified health professional to set rehabilitation goals. Because an injury impacts all areas of your being, the goals that you create should take into account physical, social, and psychological aspects. Remember to set both long-term and short-term goals which should be SMART (Taylor & Taylor, 1997).

     SMART goals refer to that fact that each goal should be:

> **S**pecific
>
> **M**easurable
>
> **A**ction-oriented
>
> **R**ealistic
>
> **T**ime-bound

     This acronym means that each of your goals should be **specific** and narrowly focused as well as able to be **measured** as to whether you successfully complete the goal or not. Furthermore, the goal should be something that you can **actively** pursue and **realistically** complete in a certain specified **time frame**. An example of a goal that encompasses all of these aspects is: I will run one mile on the track in under six minutes before April 1st. It is specific and narrowly focused as one mile in a certain time and it can be measured as to whether or not you reach your goal of six minutes. In addition, it is action-oriented as you are taking steps to achieve it, it should be realistic for yourself personally, and it is time-bound by stating that the goal is to complete it by the deadline of April 1st.

     Additionally, goals should be self-determined and modified with the help of your athletic trainer, physical therapist, or other health care professional in order to coordinate physical, social, and psychological goals during the rehabilitation process. Goal setting helps you understand the importance of rehabilitation exercises and be able to monitor your effort and success. It also provides optimal challenges, gives you a sense of being in control, and provides a sense of accomplishment. Reaching a goal can bring you joy and build self-confidence as you measure up the small successes along the way to the ultimate success; completing rehabilitation and returning to your sport or life-style.

When setting a goal it should be something you personally would like to achieve. You should also take responsibility and ownership of the goal. Seek reinforcement and support from others when creating and pursuing your goals. Telling others about your goals will increase the likelihood that you will stay on track and keep pursuing those goals. It is also important to recognize that goal setting is a process and effective goal setting occurs in three phases: planning of the goal, implementation of effort to accomplish the goal, and evaluation of the outcome. The following chart further explains the three phases of goal setting.

Planning	Set and clarify your goal, develop strategy for achievement, plan for potential setbacks. Identify specifically what you need to do to accomplish your goal and when you need to accomplish it by. Make sure that your goal is SMART
Implementation	Take steps toward the goal. Put your goals into action, monitor goals, document progress and record set-backs as well as how you overcame those setbacks
Evaluation	Monitor your progress. Document feedback on progress and accomplishments including self-evaluation and feedback from others. Evaluate outcome of your goal and begin setting new goals

Also to keep in mind is that there are different types of goals and you should strive to vary the types of goals that you set. Three main types of goals are **performance goals, process goals, and outcome goals**. A chart explaining the differences is as follows:

Type of Goal	What They Focus On	Under Your Control?	Example
Performance Goal	Personal improvement in a certain area where you wish to gain mastery or expertise	Yes	Increasing the range of motion of your injured joint 20 degrees more by a certain date.
Process Goal	Specific actions needed to perform well	Yes	Completing all of the exercises set forth by your athletic trainer every day.
Outcome Goal	Results of a task	Not completely. Outside influences are compounding factors.	Getting back to your sport post-rehabilitation before next season

Goal setting is very important for all areas of your life, not solely in rehabilitation. It provides you with motivation and something to strive toward. **Long-term goals** are those which are usually an end result goal, often outcome goals, and are those you wish to accomplish over a longer period of time (such as returning fully and safely back to your sport after rehabilitation), whereas **short-term goals** are those you wish to accomplish in the near future (in a day or week/couple of weeks) and are often process goals or performance goals. Your short-term goals should be created to help you reach your long-term goal. Make a list of some long term goals and short term goals that you would like to accomplish in various aspects of your life, including rehabilitation. Identify each of these as a performance goal, a process goal, or an outcome goal. Next, write down active steps that you can take to aid you in reaching that goal. Use the goal planning worksheet on the next few pages as an outline to help you plan out each goal and then track those goals on the goal implementation and evaluation worksheet that follows the goal planning worksheet.

Goal Setting Planning Worksheet

This worksheet is designed to help you plan out your long-term and short-term goals as well as active steps that will help you to reach those goals. Use the worksheet on the following pages to help you plan out one long-term goal with three short-term goals designed to aid you in reaching the long-term goal. Then, plan out multiple steps that you can actively take in order to assist you in reaching each one of those goals. Be as specific as possible and take ownership of your goals in order to be committed. Your long term goal should be something you personally want to achieve. Make copies of these pages as needed to help you in your planning stage if you have more goals that you would like to accomplish. Make sure that each goal you set is SMART!

Long-term Goal:

_____

_____

_____

Why this long-term goal is SMART:

Specific:

_____

Measureable:

_____

Action Oriented:

_____

Realistic:

_____

Time-Bound:

_____

What active steps will I take to reach this goal?

1. _____
2. _____
3. _____

Short-term Goal #1:

_____

_____

_____

Why this short-term goal #1 is SMART:

Specific:

_____

Measureable:

_____

Action Oriented:

_____

Realistic:

_____

Time-Bound:

_____

What active steps will I take to reach this goal?

1. _____
2. _____
3. _____

Short-term Goal #2:

_____

_____

_____

Why this short-term goal #2 is SMART:

Specific:

_____

Measureable:

_____

Action Oriented:

_____

Realistic:

_____

Time-Bound:

_____

What active steps will I take to reach this goal?

    1. _____

    2. _____

    3. _____

Short-term Goal #3:

_____

_____

_____

Why this short-term goal #3 is SMART:

Specific:

_____

Measureable:

_____

Action Oriented:

_____

Realistic:

_____

Time-Bound:

_____

What active steps will I take to reach this goal?

    1. _____

    2. _____

    3. _____

Short-term Goal #4:

_____

_____

_____

Why this short-term goal #4 is SMART:

Specific:

_____

Measureable:

_____

Action Oriented:

_____

Realistic:

_____

Time-Bound:

_____

What active steps will I take to reach this goal?

    1. _____

    2. _____

    3. _____

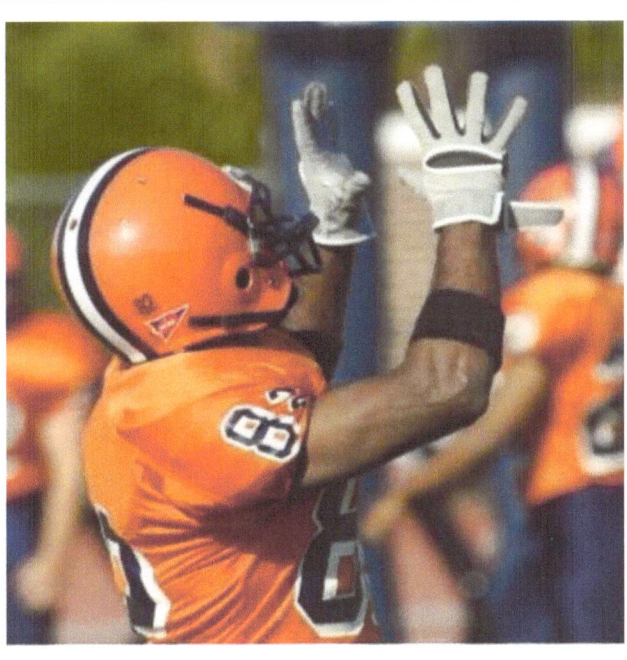

Never Stop Reaching For Your Goal

Goal Setting Implementation and Evaluation Worksheet

Use the activity log on the bottom of this page and on the next page to monitor your progress in reaching each of your goals by noting when you implement active steps toward that goal and by evaluating your progress. Track your progress toward your goal regularly on the worksheet provided. Make copies of the form to fill out for each of the goals you have outlined on the previous pages. Make any additional notes about your progress and how you feel in your journal.

GOAL (long-term or short-term):

_____

_____

Active Steps To Take Toward Goal:

_____

_____

_____

Date/Day/ Time	What I Did and How I Implemented It	How I Felt About It	Was I Successful in Implementing it?	Feedback from Others

Date/Day/ Time	What I Did and How I Implemented It	How I Felt About It	Was I Successful in Implementing it?	Feedback from Others

Psychological Relaxation Techniques

Relaxation is an important aspect in managing stress, including the stress of your injury. Psychological relaxation techniques are helpful in coping with your injury both physically and psychologically. In utilizing such exercises you can learn to better manage pain, cope with stress, and improve your psychological well-being through rehabilitation. Some relaxation techniques include **diaphragmatic breathing, stress release imagery, relaxation imagery, and progressive neuromuscular relaxation**. These can be helpful in any aspect of your life, but specifically over the course of your rehabilitation when you feel anxious, tense, stressed, or have negative feelings. While you can perform these exercises on your own by memorizing the script or guide for the technique, it is much more effective when first implementing them if you have someone read the script to you so that you can close your eyes, relax your mind, and focus all of your attention on the psychological relaxation technique at hand. A brief overview of these techniques is provided in the table below along with guided scripts for the individual exercises on the following pages.

Diaphragmatic Breathing	Focusing on the movement of the diaphragm as an accessory respiration muscle with slow controlled breathing
Stress Release Imagery	Using mental imagery to imagine stress, tension, and weight physically leaving your muscles and your body
Relaxation Imagery	Incorporating a relaxing and calming mental experience using as many senses as possible to relax and soothe the body and mind
Progressive Neuromuscular Relaxation	The progressive tensing and relaxing of muscles throughout the body as a way of releasing stress and tension

Diaphragmatic Breathing

Diaphragmatic breathing is the most valuable component in psychological relaxation interventions. This is due to the fact that it is involved in all other relaxation exercises and you must have a concrete understanding of and practice in diaphragmatic breathing before you can attempt any other relaxation techniques.. The diaphragm is the most efficient muscle of breathing because your abdominal muscles help move the diaphragm to give you more power to empty the air out of your lungs. The diaphragm is a large, dome-shaped muscle located at the base of the lungs. When you inhale your diaphragm contracts and moves downward, increasing the space in your chest for your lungs to expand as they fill up with oxygen. When you exhale your diaphragm relaxes and moves upward, reducing the space in your chest for your lungs and helping you to force the air out of your lungs. Actively engaging this muscle this muscle while breathing helps you to:

- **Strengthen the diaphragm**
- **Decrease the work of breathing by slowing your breathing rate**
- **Decrease oxygen demand**
- **Use less effort and energy to breathe**

When breathing normally, most people do not engage in diaphragmatic breathing. Instead, they use their chest muscles to expand and contract to inhale and exhale. In doing so, the diaphragm is constricted in movement and, over time, the diaphragm weakens causing it to lose its ability to move through its entire potential range of motion. When the diaphragm is unable to move through its entire potential range of motion through inhalation and exhalation, the quality of your breathing suffers as well as your voice, and eventually your health and well-being suffer as well.

Diaphragmatic Breathing Exercise

Use the following exercise to practice diaphragmatic breathing:

(Adapted from: Cleveland Clinic Health System, 2005)

1. Lie on your back on a flat surface with your knees bent, or sit comfortably in a chair with your knees bent and your body fully relaxed. You can have your eyes open or closed, whichever you are more comfortable with.

2. Place your hands loosely on your stomach just below your rib cage. This will allow you to feel your diaphragm move as you breathe.

3. Breathe in slowly and deeply through your nose so that your stomach moves out against your hand as your diaphragm contracts. Only your stomach should move as you breathe. Focus on not expanding your chest, as your chest should not move.

4. Now, tighten your stomach muscles and exhale slowly through your mouth, letting your stomach fall inward as you exhale. Feel your hand fall as your stomach deflates and your diaphragm moves upward into the chest cavity

- Make sure to control your breathing, keeping it slow and steady. This takes a lot of practice!

- For full continued relaxation, practice this technique often for about 5-10 minutes at a time and note the differences that you feel mentally or by writing them down in your journal. Challenge yourself to try to perform this technique daily throughout the course of your physical rehabilitation.

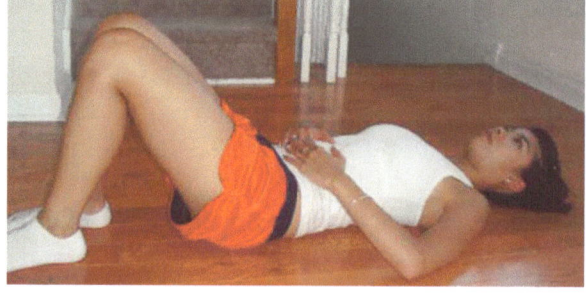

Stress Release Imagery Technique

(Adapted from: Taylor & Taylor, 1997)

- Sit or lay down in a very relaxed and comfortable position with your eyes closed. Take a couple slow deep breaths to clear your mind in through your nose and out through your mouth. Imagine that there is very heavy cement throughout your entire body. From the top of your head to your ends of your toes, your entire body feels extremely heavy, like it is stuck into the place where you are sitting or laying.

- Take a long, slow, diaphragmatic, deep breath, allowing your stomach to rise fully as you inhale through your nose and fall while you exhale slowly through your mouth.

- Now, start to let that cement go and feel the weight drain from your body starting at the top of your head as you begin to feel very relaxed. Your head starts feeling very free and the weight begins leaving your face and continuing slowly down your neck. Feel the tension leave your jaw, neck, and shoulders as you continue to breathe deeply, concentrating on your stomach rising and falling as you begin to feel more and more relaxed.

- As the weight from the cement leaves your muscles, your body begins to feel lighter and free. The weight continues to drain from your shoulders, to your upper arms, to your wrists and out through your fingertips. Allow all of the weight in your upper body and arms to leave through your fingertips as you continue to breathe slowly and deeply, in through your nose and out through your mouth. All of the weight is now lifted from your entire upper body, as it is no longer cemented in place and you feel freer and more relaxed.

- The weight from the cement is now moving through your lower body, down your back and abdominals as every muscle it passes becomes more relaxed and loose. As it passes your lower back and stomach you feel your stomach rise and fall with your deep diaphragmatic breathing. The weight begins to drain down your legs. Your thighs begin to feel heavy as all of the weight drains down them and into your lower legs. As the weight keeps draining down your body it travels down through your calves and into your feet as your thighs and lower legs feel free and relaxed. All of the heavy weight from the cement left in your body is now pooling in your feet and as it keeps draining it goes out through the tips of your toes as your body becomes free of all of the weight and all of the tension.

- Finally, all of the cement is out of your body as you lay there concentrating on your breathing, feeling extremely relaxed and comfortable, deeply inhaling slowly in through your nose and out through your mouth, feeling your stomach rise and fall. You no longer feel cemented in place, you feel light and free. You are fully relaxed. Continue breathing slowly and deeply feeling each breath go in and out.

Relaxation Imagery Technique

- Sit or lay in a comfortable position, concentrating on your diaphragmatic breathing in through your nose and out through your mouth. Feel your stomach rise with every inhalation and fall with every exhalation.

- Close your eyes and relax, let all thoughts escape your mind. Take five deep diaphragmatic breaths to clear your mind completely.

- Imagine that you are on a beach at sunset sitting in a comfortable chair. It is peaceful and quiet. You can see the horizon over the water as the sky begins to turn colors. You can feel the warm, soft sand under your feet and the wind blowing coolly on your face. You can faintly taste the salt water as you smell the ocean water in the air. No one else is on the beach and you feel content to be all alone. You can see and hear the waves crashing in front of you as you watch the white crests of the waves slowly rolling in to the shoreline and back out again.

- Now, as the waves roll in onto the shore take a deep breath in through your nose. Imagine all of the stress from your life rolling in with the waves. Every bit of your stress rolls in with the waves as you continue focusing on the salt water, the waves, the horizon, the setting sun, the cool breeze, and the warm sand.

- As the waves roll back out to the ocean let your breath completely out, and all of your stress is now being washed out to sea with the waves. As the waves drift further away, so does your stress.

- Breathe in sync with the waves, inhale through your nose feeling your stomach rise as the waves wash in on the shoreline, and exhale out through your mouth feeling your stomach fall as the wave washes all of your stress far out to sea. Allow all other thoughts to escape your mind as you focus on the beach, the water, and the roll of the waves slowly in and slowly back out.

- Continue to breathe in and out with the waves, concentrating only on the beach and the flow of the water as you feel more relaxed with each breath, having all of the stress from your life leave your body and free your mind.

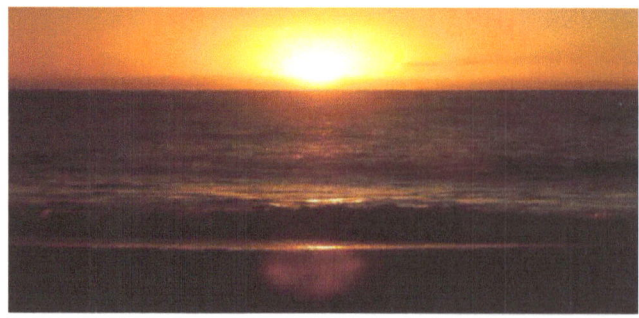

Progressive Neuromuscular Relaxation Technique

(Adapted from Glassman, 2007)

Sit or lay in a comfortable position, concentrating on your diaphragmatic breathing in through your nose and out through your mouth, feeling your stomach rise as you inhale and fall with as you exhale. **When following this script avoid tensing the injured area!!! Skip the step involving the location of your injury!** If anything causes you pain while you are completing this exercise, stop immediately.

1. To begin, feel all of the tension in your body. Acknowledge the differences in tension in different areas. Recognize where the tension is most concentrated and focus on each area.
2. Scrunch your toes and point your feet downward. Hold as tight as you can for 5 seconds, 1- 2- 3- 4- 5, and relax. Take a deep breath. Feel the difference between the tense and relaxed state.
3. Now, tighten your lower legs, knees, and thighs. Tense both of your legs as hard as you can, feeling the tension in every muscle as you contract, making your legs as straight and as stiff as possible. Hold for 5 seconds, 1- 2- 3- 4- 5, and relax, taking a slow and deep breath in through your nose and out through your mouth. Feel how relaxed your legs now are.
4. Next, tense your lower back, buttocks, abdominals, and pelvic area. Feel the difference in the tension as you squeeze tighter and tighter. Hold for 5 seconds, 1- 2- 3- 4- 5, and relax.
5. Tense your hands, lower arms, elbows, and upper arms. Feel the tension grow tighter in your fingers and hands as you make a fist and straighten your arms as hard as you can. Hold this for 5 seconds, 1- 2- 3- 4- 5, and relax. Feel the difference between the tense and relaxed state as you take a slow deep breath.
6. Now, tighten the upper back. Make your upper back and shoulders as tight as you can. Squeeze your shoulder blades together and squeeze your elbows down to your sides. Feel the tension as your shoulder and upper back muscles contact hard against the floor or your chair. Hold for 5 seconds, 1- 2- 3- 4- 5, and relax, taking a deep breath as you release.
7. Shrug your shoulders now, as though you trying to touch your shoulders to your ears. Hold for 5 seconds and feel the tension, 1- 2- 3- 4- 5, and now relax noting the difference in your body between the tensed and relaxed state.
8. Tense the neck as tight as you can, clinching your jaw to hold the tension. Feel it in your jaw and in your neck. Hold for 5 seconds 1-2-3-4-5, and release. Feel the difference between the tense and relaxed state as you continue to breathe deeply in through your nose and out through your mouth.
9. Now tighten all of the muscles in your entire head. Make a scowl on your face with your eye brows and purse your lips so that you feel the tension in all your facial muscles. Feel the tension in your eyebrow muscles as you tighten your face. Hold for 5 seconds, 1- 2- 3- 4- 5, and then relax.
10. Afterwards, open your mouth as wide as possible and raise your eye brows as high as you can. Hold this again for 5 seconds, feeling the difference 1-2-3-4-5. Then relax completely, taking a deep breath in and letting it go back out.
11. Now, try to tense every muscle in your whole body all at once. Hold it, feel the tension everywhere. Find any remaining tension and target it. Hold it as tight as you can for 5 seconds, 1-2-3-4-5. Now relax. Take several slow, deep diaphragmatic breaths in through your nose and out through your mouth. Feel the relaxation.
12. Continue sitting or lying for a few minutes, feeling the relaxation flowing through your body. Notice the difference of the relaxation in your muscles from before you began the exercise to now after you have completed it.
13. When you want to get up, count backward from five to one. You should feel relaxed, renewed, and refreshed, wide awake and calm, and ready to continue your day, 5- 4- 3- 2- 1.

Need More? What To Do If This Book Is Not Enough

This book is by no means the only resource that you should use in your psychological rehabilitation from injury. Find educational materials and techniques that work for you personally to help cope with and psychologically rehabilitate from your injury. Some athletes find it very helpful to speak to a sport psychologist about what they are experiencing mentally as they rehabilitate from their injury. A sport psychologist is an excellent resource and would also be a great person to speak with and discuss your answers and journal responses from the sections of this book. They can guide you as to what your answers and worksheets may tell you about yourself and your rehabilitation process.

Tips on Where to Look for a Sport Psychologist:

- Ask your athletic trainer if your school employs a sport psychologist or, if not, how you may be able to contact one.

- Visit a local university that employs a sport psychologist and ask to set up a private meeting.

- Go online and look for sport psychologists in your local area by typing "sport psychologist + your area or zip code" into a search engine.

- Find your state's psychological association online.

- Go to the Association for Applied Sport Psychology (AASP) website at appliedsportpsych.org/. Next, look for the certified consultant finder link to find a sport psychologist in your area.

Closing Letter to the Injured Athlete:

Dear Athlete,

As you have now completed *Return to Play: Guide to the Mental Aspects of Rehabilitation for Injured Athletes*, I hope that you have a better understanding of the psychological rehabilitation process and how it can be used in conjunction with the physical rehabilitation process to get you to a maximal level of readiness to return to your sport post-injury.

In this book, we went over your own personal roles in rehabilitation, as well as what you can control and what you can not in the rehabilitation process to give you a better understanding that there are many things that you may want to control but that you must realize are beyond your power to do so. We also discussed how to assess your perceived self-identity and how to determine your own level of athletic identity. Throughout rehabilitation, it is important to keep this in mind to try to maintain your level of athletic identity or to find other aspects of your self-identity that you can explore more throughout your injury rehabilitation process. Through the sections of cognitive appraisal as well as stress and burn out, we identified how the injury itself makes you feel, your own perceived strengths and weaknesses in various areas, and how other aspects of your life may be impacting your rehabilitation process without you even knowing it. Finally, and perhaps most importantly, we went over guidelines of how you can better manage the physical rehabilitation process and psychological rehabilitation process by incorporating psychological relaxation techniques. Feel free to revisit previous sections that have helped you as you complete your rehabilitation and continue to practice the psychological skills that you have learned, not just in rehabilitation but in your everyday life.

Now, it is up to you to get as much out of the rehabilitation process as you can both physically and psychologically. Seek the help of others as forms of social support. Remember to keep in mind that there are many types of social support including listening social support, emotional social support, educational social support, as well as numerous other kinds. No one person can provide all types of social support to you that you need and it is important that you actively seek it from multiple sources. I hope that this manual has helped you in psychologically rehabilitating from your injury and has aided in the rehabilitation process to get you back to your sport as quickly and as safely as possible.

Sincerely,

Kathleen Kickish, MS, ATC, LAT

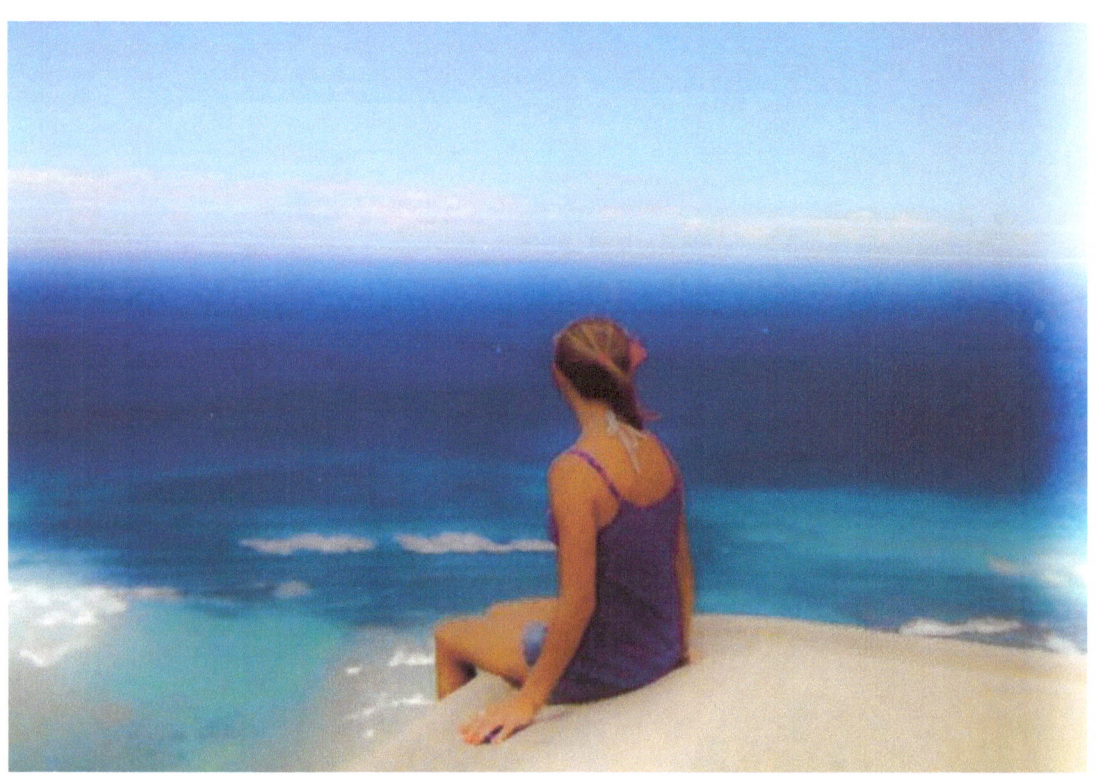

Resources

This resource section is meant to serve a dual purpose. The first purpose is to acknowledge the base of literature from which the information for this book was taken. The second purpose is to serve as a list for additional information on the subject of psychological response to injury and the psychological rehabilitation process of the injured athlete

Beck, L., Bridges, D., Gould, D., & Udry, E. (1997). Down but not out: Athletes responses to season ending injuries. *Journal of Sport and Exercise Psychology, 19,* 229-248

Brewer, B. W., & Cornelius, A. E. (2001). Norms and factorial invariance of the Athletic Identity Measurement Scale. *Academic Athletic Journal, 16,*103–113

Brough, P., & Oliver, J. (2002). Cognitive appraisal, negative affectivity, & psychological well- being. *New Zealand Journal of Psychology, 31* (1), 2-7

Cleveland Clinic Health System. (2005). *Diaphragmatic breathing.* Retrieved December 1, 2008 from Cleveland Clinic Health System's Web site:

http://www.cchs.net/health/health-info/docs/2400/2409.asp?index=9445&pflag=1

Fevre, M.L., Kolt, G.S., & Matheny, J. (2003). Eustress, distress, and interpretation in occupational stress. *Journal of Managerial Psychology, 18* (7), 726-744

Glassman, S.K. (2007). *Progressive neuromuscular relaxation (PNR).* Retrieved December 1, 2008 from Glassman Psychological Services' Web site: http://www.glassmanpsyd.com/progressive-neuromuscular-rela/

Griffith, K.A., & Johnson K.A. (2002). *Athletic identity and life roles of division I and division III collegiate athletes (pdf).* Retrieved December 1, 2008:

http://murphylibrary.uwlax.edu/digital/jur/2002/griffith-johnson.pdf

Heil, J. (1995) *Psychology of sport injury.* Champaign, IL: Human Kinetics Publishers

Holmes, T.H., & Rahe, R.H. (1967). Social readjustment rating scale. *Journal of Psychosomatic Research*, 11, 213-218.

Kubler-Ross, E. (1969). *On death and dying.* New York: Touchtone Publishers

Mummery, K., Perry, C., & Schofield, G. (2004). *Bouncing back: the role of coping style, social support, and self-concept in reliance of sport performance.* Retrieved September 16, 2010 from Athletic Insight: The Online Journal of Sport Psychology Web site:

http://wwwathleticinsight.com/Vol61ss3/BouncingBack.htm

Pargman, D. (2007). *Psychological bases of sport injuries.* Morgantown, WV: Fitness Information Technology

Taylor, J., & Taylor, S. (1997). *Psychological approaches to sports injury rehabilitation.* Gaithersburg, MD: Aspen Publishers

Susic, P. (1999). *Personality types A, B, C, and disease.* Retrieved December 1, 2008 from St. Louis Psychologists and Counseling Information and Referral Web site: \

http://www.psychtreatment.com/personality_type_and_disease.htm

All About the Author and Acknowledgements

Hello! My name is Kathy Kickish and I am a life-long athlete. Through the years, I have participated in a variety of sports including softball, track and field, soccer, field hockey, lacrosse, crew, basketball, cheerleading, and Tae Kwon Do. During participation in those sports, I was a bit of an "accident prone" athlete due to my aggressive nature and hard work on and off the field. That being said, in high school I became well acquainted with our high school's athletic trainer, who sparked my interest in the field of Athletic Training.

I obtained my Bachelor's of Science degree in Athletic Training from The George Washington University and passed the Board of Certification exam to become a National Athletic Trainer's Association Certified Athletic Trainer (ATC) in 2009. Although I was proficient in the physical rehabilitation of the injured athlete, I could not help but notice the psychological aspects of injury that impacted the athletes I worked with as they went through their physical rehabilitation. Therefore, I went on to pursue a graduate degree in the field of Sport and Exercise Psychology. I earned my Master's of Science degree in May of 2011 from Temple University's Psychology of Movement program, where I combined my knowledge of the physical rehabilitation process of injury with the psychological response to injury and the psychological rehabilitation process. Since graduating, I have obtained licensure as a certified athletic trainer in the states of New Jersey and Pennsylvania and am currently employed as a full time athletic trainer for NovaCare Rehabilitation.

I would like to thank Dr. Amanda Visek, a professor at The George Washington University, whom I had the pleasure of studying under during the final year of my undergraduate degree. In Dr. Visek's Psychology of Injury class, not only was my interest sparked in the subject of the psychological response to injury, but I also began the psychological rehabilitation book that you are now reading. I would also like to thank Dr. Michael Sachs, my adviser and professor at Temple University, who furthered my interest in the field of sport and exercise psychology, as well as guided me into the narrow focus of combining my knowledge of the physical rehabilitation process with my interest in the psychological aspects of injury. It is to them that I owe my completion of this book! I would also like to give a big thank you to SammyNicks Photography for donating many great sports photos for the creation of this book and to the many individuals who professionally or personally gave help, feedback, criticisms, and encouragement. Thank you all so very much!